REFLECTIONS
WITHIN MY MIND

Reflections

WITHIN MY MIND

Michelle Anneliese Benvenuto

Table of Contents

REFLECTIONS WITHIN MY MIND

Have you ever looked into a mirror only to find your reflection completely unrecognizable? Or asked yourself 'how did I get here, and where am I going'? Lately I find myself asking these exact questions. The confusion I'm facing is that I don't think I know the answers. Or, maybe in my subconscious mind I do.

I'll try to give an explanation by flickering back into my mind's eye certain events in my life. By unscrambling those reflections within my mind this may help me to explain, so as to be understood. I often wonder what my life would have been like if those events didn't take place. You can only wonder.

I'll have to take a trip down memory lane to around 30 years ago when I had not a care in the world. I was just a teenager, but in such a hurry to be an adult. I always thought being an adult would be so great, and how good it would be to be able to do what I wanted, when I wanted.

Wrong. Wrong. Wrong.

When I was at high school, I was known to have a lot of friends. I was a good, honest, trustworthy student, easy going, with my head full of dreams about my future. I always wanted to help people and I wanted to travel the world. I also loved children and was considering teaching. My thoughts of either being a travel hostess or teaching played back and forward in my mind. I was so young, and I thought I had all the time in the world. But don't we all. I'm in my later life now, and yet it seems like yesterday the decisions about my life were all so different. Life can be so unpredictable, so I learned.

October 1981, I was married at seventeen years of age (unfortunately without my parents blessing, due to my age) to a handsome Italian, who I deeply loved. Still do. He was twenty-two years old. At eighteen I had my first child, a daughter. As I had always loved children, particularly newborns, I took to motherhood without a hitch. I adored my baby girl. Twenty-two months later I gave birth to my first boy, my husband's pride and joy. Another two years passed, and I gave birth to my little princess. She was like a porcelain doll, so fragile and delicate. Then, you guessed it, two years later my second son was born. My little man.

I had four children in a space of 6 years. I was now aged twenty-three. I loved being a wife and mother. My children are very precious to me, still are, even though my baby is now married. In fact, they all are. Now the oldest two have children themselves. Two girls to my first daughter, and a daughter to my oldest son. That's three beautiful granddaughters.

At twenty-six, I had a miscarriage which totally devastated me. You never really get over something like that. It wasn't the first time either. I also had one before my first daughter was born. It's a hard loss to deal with. You learn to dull your mind so you can cope. Often telling yourself 'it wasn't meant to be, it's for the best'. It doesn't stop you however, thinking of how your son or daughter would have looked, or what sort of personality they would have had.

Anyway, now being a full-time mum and wife, I kept my days busy. I never pursued a secular career as being a mum was fulltime work for me. I also have a very old-fashioned husband, who had very strong opinions about the duties of a mother and wife. He expected me to be at home and attending to the household. I didn't mind though.

I had a lot to keep me busy. I had a lot to do teaching scripture classes, volunteering at the canteen, helping teachers with reading, craft, and generally where there was a need at the public school. I even attended some of the children's excursions, which they loved. I also took up selling Avon as a hobby and that helped me feel a bit independent.

As to my duties as a housewife, I was a perfectionist in this area, which sometimes was exhausting. Yes, I was one of those fanatical mums cleaning continually into the late evening, hanging up washing at midnight and vacuuming three times a day. I know this got on everyone's nerves, but I couldn't help it. I was taught as a child that cleanliness was next to godliness.

I remember when my grandmother would come to visit, how I would have to jump out of bed at 6 o'clock in the morning, make my bed, and help my mother get the house in tip top shape before leaving for school. This applied to my brothers also. I guess it stuck, which I suppose wasn't a bad thing.

Now back to my children. Once my children went to high school, I became a little concerned. My eldest daughter was fine, she was an A student and flew through high school without too many problems. But my boys had learning problems, particularly my eldest son, being diagnosed with ADHD when he was in the fourth grade. My second daughter was very scared and shy about going to high school. She developed a social phobia and didn't like to leave my side. (There was a reason for this, but I'll clarify that later).

Anyway, I then decided to teach my children myself. I contacted The Board of Studies and asked what I would have to do to teach my children. A middle-aged man from the Board of Studies came and interviewed me to see if I was capable of such a task. I had to have individual programs for each child, which I did. So, I taught three of my children at home, instead of them going to a public high school. At the age of 15 they all had jobs.

It was not easy, but I don't regret it for a minute. Particularly the expression on my daughter's face made it all worthwhile. The relief she felt was indescribable. Her anguish simply disappeared, making her feel safe and protected. Isn't that a parent's role? For this reason, I believe I did the right thing even though many people criticized me for it.

My eldest son is now a Pest Technician. He had to do several courses to be fully qualified for this profession. I'm very proud of his accomplishments. He's had to work very hard to achieve this. He is also the father of a precious little girl. He also got divorced two years ago but has now found his lifelong partner. He's very happy and that's all I care about. She's a lovely young woman who adores my son. I wish them every happiness.

My youngest son works full time for Kellogg's. He is a persistent hard worker and is still very young. He has a lot of potential and ambition. He's married and lives next door to us and he too is very happy with his partner, who is currently completing a Hair Dressing Apprenticeship. (Free hair colouring for me!)

As for my eldest daughter she is now going through the process of becoming a nurse, or maybe even a doctor. As well as being a mother of two beautiful girls, she is very much in love with her husband.

My second daughter didn't want a secular career. She just wanted to become a wife and mother, and my full-time personal carer. Funny enough she became my full-time care giver at age sixteen and married when she turned twenty to her childhood sweetheart. She was ridiculed by some for her decision to work as her mother's carer, saying that it wasn't a real job, but she didn't care. It was her greatest desire, and she has been working as my carer for 6 years now, as well as a loyal companion.

I can hear you asking why a 16-year-old girl (at the time) would need or want to be her mother's carer. Particularly, when her mother was such a perfectionist and kept herself so active.

As I stated before, life is unpredictable, sometimes we have to deal with situations beyond our control. I speak from experience, believe me.

A NIGHT THAT CHANGED EVERYTHING

One night my whole world changed. I remember it clearly. Sunday, December 27, 1992. I have never spoken of it in detail, but I think it's time I did. I want to share what happened to me and the effect it had on my family.

We had just spent the weekend at my in-laws. I was recovering from a recent operation. Six weeks prior, the doctors discovered I had a cyst on my right ovary. So,

I had it removed. They couldn't save the ovary, but a woman can survive with one, so I didn't worry too much. It wasn't as though I was planning to have any more children. Because the cyst was quite a good size, I needed six weeks recovery and that's why we were at my in-laws for the weekend.

I had a little headache that morning. I remember taking some Disprin (also known as Asprin). After lunch, we set off for home. We wanted to get back early. The children had school in the morning. They were all attending primary school at that time. Their ages were 10, 8, 6, and 4 years old.

My in-laws lived in the western suburbs, and we had a 2-hour trip home to the central coast. On our way home, I wanted to visit my father's gravesite. He had passed away ten years earlier, on the 4th of August 1982, just six weeks before my 1st child was born. He was only forty years old when he died.

My parents were divorced when I was 3 years old. I still had a relationship with my father though. My mother never stopped me from having a relationship with him. I thank her for that. I always knew who my father was and would see him on school holidays and so forth. It ripped a hole in my heart when he passed away and I cried excessively. He would have made such a good grandfather. He was so easy going and had a good sense of humour.

The last time I saw him, he was very sick, and very weak. He had Cancer and he knew he was dying. He also told me not to come back to see him. I didn't understand why at the time. He wanted me to remember him at his best. He was also worried that me seeing him like that would be too distressing to the baby I was carrying. Life can sometimes be so unfair, but there's nothing you or I can do about it. You just have to play with the cards you have been dealt.

As I sat a while beside my father's resting place, I would talk to him, telling him how the children were and so forth. I know he couldn't hear me, as I don't believe in heaven or hell. I believe we're just sleeping when we die. In a peaceful state, no longer able to feel any pain. This brought me great comfort, because I know my papa's illness was very painful at the end. Still, it helped me cope with his passing by talking to him. When I was able to say goodbye to my papa, we made our 2-hour trip home. I was quite exhausted, feeling a little emotional (as I normally am after reminiscing of happier times with my papa).

It was now early evening approximately 8.30pm. I had just put the children to bed. I was feeling a little tired. That Disprin I had taken earlier in the day really didn't help. So, I thought I would have a shower and go to bed. Hopefully a good night sleep is all I needed. Just as I was about to go to bed, the phone rang. It was a friend of my husbands. It would have been around 9.30pm. As I handed him the phone I gave him a quick kiss on the cheek, checked on the children (that were already tucked into bed) and headed off to bed myself.

I remember waking up to go to the bathroom. My husband had just come to bed. I checked the children on the way back to my bedroom. As soon as my head hit the pillow, I felt a very strange sensation come over my whole body, the best way I could describe it was like, a wave, very disoriented, almost drunk like. The room was beginning to spin. It was starting to concern me, so I went to tell my husband, who was facing away from me. I couldn't speak - just strange sounds were coming from my mouth, that even I couldn't understand. My right arm then locked stiff, in front of my face. I tried to unbend it, but it wouldn't go. I was able to get my husband's attention finally by kicking him with my left leg. Bewildered by these events, I couldn't understand what was happening to me. My husband kept asking me "what's wrong, what's wrong". I could only make grunting sounds. I was unable to answer him. I was trying to sit up but kept falling back down.

My husband went to turn on the light. I'll never forget the look on his face; it was that of sheer horror.

There must have been quiet a commotion being made on our part, because as I looked across the bedroom, I noticed my eldest daughter with my youngest son standing in the doorway. They looked extremely frightened. At this point I was starting to go in and out of consciousness. I remember seeing two paramedics and them asking me questions. I knew the answers to the questions, but I just couldn't speak. I knew something was terribly wrong, I just didn't know what it was.

I could hear my husband's voice, in the background, and I do recall being carried out to the ambulance and my husband accompanying me. The whole time I was just worried about the children. Asking myself, "who's looking after the children?"

I was getting myself into a bit of panic, as it's
not like my husband to leave the children
alone in the house, particularly at night. I
received a large needle in the ambulance,
and I remember the paramedic cutting the
top of my nightie. I was upset that he cut it, it
was my favourite one. Then I don't remember
anything after that. I was unconscious. It was
about 10pm when all of this took place.

I awoke days later, hearing the muffled
sounds of my husband's voice in the
background. I looked across the room. I could
just make out that there was someone talking
to him. A doctor and two of our dearest
friends. I didn't stay awake for long. I would
just open my eyes from time to time. I had no
concept of time at that moment. I wasn't

aware that I had been in an induced state of sleep for 48 hours. It took all of my energy to stay awake for 5 or 10 minutes.

When I was able to wake up more fully, I noticed that I was hooked up to a lot of machinery. I didn't understand why I had a tube placed down my throat either. I wanted to get someone's attention, but I was unable to move. Confined to bed hooked up to all this machinery isn't a good sign, I thought to myself. When was somebody going to let me know what's going on? I no sooner finished that thought than a doctor with a concerned look on his face was coming towards me. I could see my husband, coming up on the other side of my bed as well. The doctor grabbed my chart and looked thoroughly through it. He stood beside me, looked at me for a moment and then asked me if I knew where I was. I didn't know. I just looked at him, as I couldn't respond. He then went to examine me by lifting my right arm. He said, "I want to see if you can hold your arm straight up in the air for me". At this point I'm thinking, of course I can. To my amazement, I could not. He held my arm up 3 times, every time it fell quickly back to the bed. I began to get upset as I still didn't know what was wrong with me.

He then went to remove the tube from my throat, pulling it out slowly, it seemed to take forever. I was astonished, that I was not choking during this procedure. He then stated, he was checking to see if my gag reflex had returned. Obviously, it hadn't. The doctor proceeded to sit next to me and said:

"Good morning, my name is Dr Denis Crimmins, and I am your doctor here at Gosford Hospital. You are In the Intensive Care Unit and have been here for a few days now." He added "Welcome back, you gave us all a bit of a scare. You will probably need to be with us for quite a while." He looked at my husband, and then back at me before continuing.

"Michelle, it seems that you've had a Cerebral Embolism, which is a blood clot. It swept through an artery inside your brain. This has caused you to be paralysed on the right side of your body. I can't tell you what your prognosis will be at this stage, only time will tell." He paused for a moment. "Do you understand?"

I must have looked confused to him because he then added. "You have had a major stroke and have managed to survive through it. You're definitely a fighter! You'll have to go through a lot of rehabilitation though, to learn how to walk and to regain all the functions of your arm again, for as long as it takes." He continued to look at me.

It was at that point I thought the doctor was completely crazy. Strokes are for elderly people. I'm only twenty-eight. He's got it all wrong, so I thought.

"I will come back and check on you tomorrow, ok?" said the doctor, before leaving my husband and I alone to absorb the news. My husband grabbed my hand telling me everything was going to be ok. He looked completely exhausted. I found out later that he had not been home since they brought me in here. He wouldn't leave my side, which was endearing but I was concerned about the children. It seemed like such a long time since I had seen them.

Meanwhile, I still had the tube down my throat, so I couldn't say anything. I was told by my husband that this tube down my throat and all this machinery is keeping me alive. It was a life support machine. Hopefully I wouldn't need it much longer.

Many thoughts were playing throughout my mind at this stage. Like, Will I ever regain my functions? Will I be my old self once more? How long would I remain in this paralysed state? How will I look after my household? The children, what about the children, and why haven't they been in to see me? All of a sudden, I began to get extremely tired. I didn't want to think about it anymore. It was too unbelievable and overwhelming for me to take in. I thought maybe I was in a bad dream, and everything would be back to normal when I woke up.

It wasn't however a bad dream, it turned out to be a cold, hard, horrible fact that I would have to accept. I was going to be in the fight of my life to regain my former self. I didn't know how long it might take, but I had to get well. I had to get back home to my children and get my life back. I was going to prove the doctor's assessment of me was totally incorrect.

My husband finally went home to get some sleep. He also had to organize the children. They had been placed in our friends care throughout this whole ordeal. They were told that mummy was very sick and would have to stay in the hospital for a while. In the meantime, they would have to stay with our friends so daddy could help the doctor's look after mummy.

When I think back now, my children must have felt so lost and confused, as I had never been away from them before. Life as we knew it was going to have a dramatic change concerning everyone in the family.

STARTING OVER FROM SCRATCH

The day finally came when those machines were turned off. That tube was then taken out of my throat. I was then asked by the doctor if I could state my full name. As I went to say my name, another word came out of my mouth.

My answer was completely irrelevant to the question I was asked. I don't know why I said that. I was now getting frustrated with myself. I seemed to have no control regarding

my thought pattern and my actual speech.
The doctor didn't seem too surprised he said
this was quite normal in stroke victims to lose
their speech for a while as the brain has been
starved of oxygen, so it takes a while for new
pathways to be made. He told me that "when
new pathways are made your speech will
return, so don't worry, I'll send you to a
speech therapist. You will start tomorrow."

He then helped me to sit up, and asked the
nurses to give assistance as he wanted to see
if I could walk across the room. The whole
time I'm thinking, what does he mean, why
wouldn't I be able to walk across the room?

It was then at that precise moment it had
finally hit me as I was asked to take a step or

two. With disbelief, my legs felt like lead, they didn't want to move, they couldn't even take a step. Why don't they walk? A two-year-old can walk, why can't I? Then I collapsed, the thought of not being able to walk was horrifying. It was with assurance I was placed back into bed. The doctor kept reassuring me:

"Don't forget it takes time for the new pathways to be made. You are still very young this can work in your favour. Most of your functions should return. We'll get you started on your rehabilitation shortly."

He then left me in the nurse's care, for the evening.

The next morning came around quickly, and I was awakened by two nurses who were going to take me for my first shower. I had been getting sponged down in bed until now, which was a little embarrassing, so this was something positive for me. I couldn't help but wonder how they were going to achieve this task, but sure enough one of the nurses brought over a waterproof wheelchair for me. They both had to lift me into the wheelchair as I still didn't have any movement in my legs.

As they were organizing the shower for me, I overheard one nurse say that under no circumstances was there a mirror to be brought in. I was never to be left unattended. I could understand them having to attend to me but couldn't understand why I couldn't have a mirror. At this point I couldn't even ask. So, I just sat there waiting to be taken into the shower. I normally don't like undressing in front of anyone as I'm extremely self-conscious, but in this case, I had no choice. Before I knew it, I was naked, wheeled into the shower, and washed.

This was quite an undignified situation to be in. I couldn't help but wonder how my husband would cope with this situation.

As the nurse finished putting a fresh gown on me an alarm went off in the next room. The nurse told me she had to attend to that call as they were understaffed and that she would be back in a moment to put me back into bed. I sat there for quite a few moments. When I looked up, I saw a mirror on the wall above the sink. I realised I hadn't seen my own face since this whole ordeal began. I wanted to see.

I couldn't help but notice the nurses had a peculiar look on their face when dealing with me. I also recall my husband reaffirming that I was 'still beautiful', so I was naturally curious to see what they weren't telling me. I tried to stretch my body upwards a little to try and catch a glimpse of myself. To my absolute horror I did just that. The right-hand side of my face had dropped severely. I saw a reflection, but it was completely unrecognizable to me. I was screaming inside. I've turned into something hideous, no wonder my husband hasn't brought the children in to see me, I thought. They wouldn't recognize me. I don't recognise me! They would be so frightened. I looked like I was deformed.

The tears built up in my eyes, tears were rolling down my cheek as I tried to understand why this had happened to me. I couldn't help but think that maybe I'd been punished for something. Why was God letting this happen to me? I considered myself to be a good person, and yet this was happening to me. It just didn't make any sense to me.

When the nurse returned, I suddenly felt extremely overwhelmed and just wanted to stay in bed and sleep the rest of the day.

That, however, I wasn't allowed to do. It was not long when my nurse returned informing me that I would try and eat my first meal. Up to now I had been fed intravenously, so I gathered this to be some form of progress on my behalf. Though my first meal would only consist of soup and jelly that a nurse had to feed to me, like a baby. I probably should have also been given a bib, as I did make a little mess, I just couldn't feel the right-hand side of my face at all. Even opening my mouth was difficult. Still, I was making progress.

Later that morning a speech therapist came to see me. She went through all the sounds of the alphabet and vowel sounds. I had to learn to talk all over again. I found this to be extremely frustrating, as I knew how to speak. It came easy in my thoughts – I just had trouble speaking my thoughts aloud. My brain and mouth were no longer in sync. I had to train it by thinking of a particular letter of the alphabet and producing the correct sound. This doesn't sound difficult to do, but it was.

I remember getting so angry with myself because I was not getting the sounds right that I burst into tears and the speech therapist had to stop the session and organized to come back the following day. I wasn't handling this situation very well. I could slowly feel myself falling into a depressed state. I was starting to doubt my own abilities.

That little voice you have in your head, the one that tells you not to give up, you can do it, keep going... it was fading out so much that I could hardly hear it.

However, I kept bringing my thoughts back to my family and something in me just plain refused to give up. I had to fight. I'm still fighting. My family didn't deserve this. They need me back as I was. I knew then what had to be done to regain myself back. Determination was starting to build inside me. The fight had just begun.

I thought learning to talk was difficult. That was nothing compared with learning to write left-handed. I used to be right-handed, like most of the population, but now since that part of my brain didn't work anymore, I had to learn to write left-handed. Again, therapists gave me sheets of letters of the alphabet, this time to trace. Joining those dots sounds easy, but it wasn't. At one stage I threw the pen and paper across the room. I couldn't believe I was no longer capable of even writing my name. I wasn't turning out to be a cooperative patient. I was starting to become angry with the world, although I was still determined to lick this.

The next few days repeated themselves with speech, writing and even learning-to-feed-my-self lessons. I had to be showered by the nurses every morning and given an injection daily in my stomach to thin my blood. I was black and blue and covered with bruising.

I remember one morning a nurse came into my room informing me that I would be taken to a hospital in Sydney where they were going to perform a special ultrasound on my throat. Also, I was to have another MRI scan. Apparently, I had one when I first arrived in hospital. They needed to do another one, as they had to wait for a week to pass by to see how much of my brain had been damaged.

I didn't see my husband that morning and I was upset, because I had no way of letting him know where I was. Still, I knew he would come to visit me, as he came every day. I also knew he would be upset and worried about me. I was just hoping that I wouldn't be too long. Within the hour I was on my way to Sydney in an ambulance. I hadn't had breakfast that morning due to the test I had to have. I didn't have to worry about going to the bathroom as I still had the catheter in me that was inserted when I arrived in hospital.

The test seemed to take forever as the hospital was understaffed due to it only being a few days into the New Year. One nurse told me, that I picked a bad time of the year to have a stroke, because a lot of the staff were on holidays. What a thing to say, I thought. As if you plan to have a stroke. She's fortunate that I wasn't able to give her a comeback. I would have had plenty to say.

Anyway, it was getting close to dinner time even though I totally missed lunch. I was hungry but I couldn't tell anyone, so I just thought I'd take a nap. Hopefully I would be back at hospital to have dinner.

I wondered how my husband was. I knew he would be anxious to see me. He has always been overprotective of me. I was imagining him pacing up and down the corridor in hospital waiting impatiently for me. I was now on the way back at least. I should have been back at the hospital for dinner, but as we were on the highway there was a call on the radio for the paramedics that a fight had broken out in a nearby jail, and there were many casualties. Then I overheard the paramedic reply to the call saying, that he was near the vicinity so he could reply to the call.

I couldn't believe it. Now here I was paralysed, not able to speak, hungry, tired, and now instead of going straight back to hospital I'm now going to a jail. What a day I'm having. Wait till husband hears about this.

Now I can think back and laugh, but at the time it was far from being funny. It was quite frightening to be parked in the driveway of a jail with sirens blazing. When the ambulance arrived, the paramedics opened the back door to get their equipment, leaving the door wide open. Why would you do that? Particularly when there's a paralysed patient in the back of the ambulance. I was so scared, I felt like I was in some bizarre dramatic motion picture or something. My imagination was getting the best of me. I was trying to keep myself calm.

They would have been gone for more than an hour when suddenly I heard footsteps. Thank goodness, the paramedics had returned and we were finally going back to hospital. I couldn't wait to see my husband and have dinner.

I arrived back at the hospital approximately 9pm. My husband was frantic. He came rushing towards me as I was being wheeled back into my room. I remember him looking closely at me. He then kissed me on my forehead and went to talk to the nurse in charge of the ward. I could still hear his voice even though I couldn't see him. He was really upset and stated they should have informed him first before they took me out of the hospital. He was talking to the nurse for quite some time.

When he came back to me, he asked me if I had eaten. I shook my head. He made sure I got something to eat, even helping me to eat it by guiding my hand to my mouth. After I had eaten and he saw that I was starting to fall asleep, he told me he would be back in the morning. As he walked away, he just gave me a smile. I couldn't but wonder how he was really doing, and how the children were.

The next morning came and after the usual routine of breakfast and shower the Doctor returned for a visit. "I hear you had quite an adventure yesterday," he said with a grin. "Let's see your chart, I think we're going to get you up and walking today." He added.

Sure enough, today was going to be my first walking lesson. The Physiotherapist and a nurse held me up on each side taking slow steps. I dragged my feet for three steps, which took 10 minutes. I couldn't do any more. I was completely exhausted as though I had just run a marathon. I felt so heavy. I had to be carried back to bed and then the Physio Therapist spoke to me about what time in the day she would come to get me. I had to practice taking those small steps every day until I was walking. No one could tell me how long it would take or even IF I WOULD BE ABLE TO WALK AGAIN.

My doctor told me I would be taken out of
Intense Care now and placed in my own
room. I could now have visitors if I wished. I
didn't really want to see anybody just yet. I
only wanted to see my children. I hadn't seen
the children for several days, although they
had given cards and drawings to their father
to give me, to make sure that I knew they
were thinking of me. There was nothing like
seeing their faces and giving them a hug.

By now, I was starting to regain a little speech
back. Enabling me now to say a few words. I
wanted desperately to be able to talk to my
children. I would go over in my mind what I
would say to them, and then practice it
aloud. I even got my Speech Therapist to help
me. It wouldn't be long before my husband

would bring the children in to see me. I don't know why I was getting so nervous, but I was. My husband told me he would bring them in the following day in the afternoon, after lunch. He had to organize to get the children as they were still staying at our friend's houses. The girls were at one place, and the boys at another. They wouldn't have to stay there much longer now that the danger period was over concerning my health.

My husband was going to be staying at home with the children now. It was the January 1993 school holidays and he had already notified his work that he was having the whole month of January off as well. Funny enough he worked as a handyman in the maintenance department for Wyong Hospital.

I have tried to recall exactly what happened concerning my first visit with my children. This is how I remember it. There were so many emotions explored from that one visit.

It was later that morning that Dr Crimmins found me. He wanted to let me know the results of my last MRI scan. He knew my family was coming to visit me after lunch and wanted to speak to me before the visit. He told me I was starting to look a lot better now than when I first arrived in hospital. Then he grabbed a chair and sat beside me. He was holding a lot of paperwork. Reading through it silently, he then looked up at me and told me the following:

"Michelle, it appears from the MRI that you have had a very severe stroke. As you can see here on the x-ray nearly the whole left side of your brain shows up black. That black part means that all that part of the brain has been damaged or died. I was hoping to have better news for you as once the brain has been damaged like this it cannot be reversed. However, that's not to say you can't make new pathways. You are only twenty-eight, so you still have youth on your side. I would recommend that you didn't have any more children though, as it could turn out to be fatal." He paused for a moment, and then he added. "As for your recovery, going by the results of your tests, it appears to be limited. You'll probably have to learn to write with your left hand, and I don't think you'll be able to do intricate work, like hand sewing or fiddly things. Be happy with the basics. It could have been a lot worse, you're lucky to be alive. I was really worried about you," he said with sincerity.

"As for your prognosis for walking..." He paused. "I honestly don't know. A lot depends on how much you want to walk. It will take some time, but you'll have to walk with an aid, either someone's arm to help you or a stick." I was trying to take this all in when my husband popped his head through my door. He had arrived with the children a little earlier than expected. The children were waiting in the corridor. As he entered the room the doctor stood up and said to me, he was going to have a quick word with my husband. They both stood outside the door and at that moment my two girlfriends walked in with my children.

My youngest daughter walked in followed by the other children. She was holding a bunch of flowers in her little hands. She looked straight at me then she looked at the bed next to mine. Looking confused she said to her father that they had the wrong room as mummy wasn't here. The other children just stood silently.

"There's mum" he said, pointing to me while he continued talking to the doctor. She looked completely puzzled. It was then I said, "It's me, mummy" and I started to cry. My own children didn't even recognize their own mother. It was my worst fear coming true. I had to try to compose myself, I didn't want to make it harder for the children than it already was.

My husband finished talking to the doctor. He put his hand out to guide my daughter to me. Her arms were stretched out as far as they could go, coming towards me with that puzzled look. My oldest daughter could see it was me, but she looked shocked to see what had happened to me, standing next to me with tears rolling down her cheek. My boys didn't say anything. They just stood quietly close to their father.

It was a rather uncomfortable situation to be in. My husband tried to make conversation to make everything ok. I was feeling very anxious, I couldn't do anything to change my appearance, and as I tried to speak, I wasn't making any sense whatsoever. I so much wanted to give them all a hug, but they seemed very unsure of me. I knew then it would take some time for the children to adjust to the way I looked.

My youngest daughter still wasn't sure that it was me and my boys were getting a little restless, so my husband took them with him to the kiosk to get me some lemonade and get them a snack. My eldest daughter however wanted to stay with me. "Come" I was able to say. She sat next to me holding my hand, saying to me repeatedly "don't worry mum, everything is going to be alright, I'll take care of you".

I think she took on my role as a mother and had to take on a lot of responsibility at her young age of 10. She didn't complain, she was a comfort to me. I didn't even have to speak it was as though she knew what I was thinking. I remember trying to tell her to cancel a dinner guest we had arranged weeks prior. I wasn't making any sense, but she turned to me and said, "it's alright mum, I told dad to cancel with them."

I just looked at her overwhelmed with tears in my eye's she knew what I was trying to say. She just sat there quietly for a short while, I remained silent, and she continued to stroke my hand.

When the rest of the family returned with my lemonade and their snacks, the boy's sat down on the floor and ate their packet of chips, and my youngest daughter gave me a drawing that she had been working on for days. It was a picture of our family and our house. We all looked so happy that it brought more tears to my eyes. I bent down and gave her a hug and said, "thank you". I placed it on my bed side table where it remained during the entire stay in hospital.

During this short visit with my children, my conviction to regain my health became overly apparent. I regained strength from deep in my soul, and I knew I would walk and talk again. Nothing would stop me I was too young to be confined to bed. My children needed their mother back, not a substitute.

The children said their goodbyes, and then they waited in the waiting room with my girlfriends as my husband wanted to talk privately for a moment to discuss the brief talk that he had with Dr Crimmins and so forth. Then he left too, and I was back to being alone again in this sterile room. I was feeling very emotional after this visit with my family. I just wanted to go to sleep. I did a lot of that.

LEARNING TO STAND ON MY OWN FEET

I was informed that my stay at Gosford Hospital would soon be coming to an end. I was going to be transferred to Wyong Hospital, which was great news to me as my husband worked there in the maintenance department as I mentioned before. It was also closer to home – only a 7-minute drive by car, so I would feel closer to my family.

I was told however, that I would be calling Wyong Hospital home for several weeks.

A few days before the transfer I had a particularly memorable day. There were many days that I had to rely on my inner voice to get me through the day, and this day was one of them. My stubborn determination got the best of me.

As I've stated before the hospital was very understaffed. I was being taken for my morning shower. I was sitting in a wheelchair in the bathroom and the nurse had just turned on the shower. She was just about to wash me when she got called to see another patient and she left me under the shower. She said she would only be a minute. So, as you can imagine here, I was left under the shower wondering how long the nurse would be. A couple of minutes had of gone by so then I thought to myself, as I looked at the soap, I can wash myself. As I went to reach for soap I fell out of my wheelchair and I couldn't, as hard as I tried, get up!

There you have it, probably my most embarrassing moment. I lay on the shower floor for at least 10 minutes before the nurse returned. Trying to scramble up into my wheelchair, wrinkled like a prune. I felt utterly helpless and humiliated and extremely embarrassed.

After the nurse picked me up and gave me a little scolding, I returned to my bed waiting for my physiotherapy to start. That day I was supposed to try and walk without the aid of any help. I didn't like my chances after that fiasco in the bathroom that morning.

Anyway, the physiotherapist came and took

me in my wheelchair to the physio room

where I was supposedly going to perform my

newfound abilities.

Sure enough, it wasn't going well. I fell down

more times than I could count. To make

things worse my stepfather appeared around

the door. I had not spoken to him for quite

some time. I didn't leave home on friendly

terms. He had moved to Queensland and

now was also divorced from my mother, who

had gone back to Germany, the place of her

birth. But he was there larger than life and I

had to deal with this situation. As I glanced

across the room, I watched him pull out a

chair and sat quietly against the wall. He gave

a small wave and just watched. I tried to pretend that he wasn't there as I felt nervous enough. I didn't want anybody to see me. I wasn't used to my condition yet and was nowhere near ready to let anybody see me like this. I didn't want anyone's pity – least of all his. I just had to grit my teeth together and proceed with my physio.

I tried as hard as I could not to look like I didn't know how to walk but when I looked at my stepfather's face it was all too apparent that he knew otherwise. He looked at me with great despair as he raised his hand over his mouth. I began to sob. I couldn't do any more and the nurse took me back to my room. My stepfather followed. He didn't say much just that he wanted to see me in person to see that I was alright, and he was sorry that this had happened to me. I think it was a bit of a shock for him to see me like that. It was still a shock for me.

He didn't stay long but I must admit it was nice of him to come. It showed me that he still cared a little for me as he did raise me as his own child from a very young age. Unfortunately, things sometimes change as we get older. I don't really have anything much to do with him now, but I still ask about him and know how he's doing. I'll always remember though, that he went out of his way to see me at Gosford Hospital. This has stayed with me and regardless of our past problems, I prefer to remember him for this kind gesture.

I had a few visitors during my stay in Gosford Hospital. Mainly different family members such as my grandmother, my mother-in-law, sisters-in-law, and so forth. All of them trying to keep composure during their short visits.

I must admit I was starting to feel like I belonged at the circus in a freak show. It was getting a little unbearable for me to receive any more visitors, so I requested no visitors except for my husband and children.

I decided this after one of my dearest friends came to see me. It wasn't easy for her to come to see me. Her father had recently passed away in hospital, so it was still emotionally hard for her to enter any hospital.

She didn't say much, and I could tell she was feeling uncomfortable. Since she was in the same religion as me, she decided to read some articles to me and relate some events that happened recently.

It was during this time I felt wetness on my legs. It was a very awkward moment for me. I had just had my catheter removed that morning and my body hadn't registered it was gone just yet. Another embarrassing moment for me, having to get a nurse called to my room to change the bed. Fancy wetting the bed at the age of twenty-eight.

After getting my bed changed, I was feeling very embarrassed and my friend could sense that, so she decided to go. She told me not to

worry about it and she would see me when I
went to Wyong Hospital. She kissed my
cheek, gave me a hug, and left.

Finally, the day came to be transferred to
Wyong Hospital. I was to go by ambulance
after lunch, which I did. I had my own room
in the Rehab Unit along with approximately
18 patients. I was of course the youngest. The
rest of the patients were fifty plus, so I was
considered to be the baby of the group. I was
in room 7, where I remained for several
weeks.

It was a nice room. I had my own television
and ensuite, and it had a pleasant view of the
grounds. This would be home to me until the
Doctors thought I was ready to leave.

I wondered how long my recovery would take. I needed to get back to life as I knew it. I also knew that it depended on me and how quickly I was able to function in the real world. I had a long way to go but was determined to do what the Doctors said, because I didn't want to be in hospital longer than I had to.

Later that afternoon, the occupational therapist came to see me. She was middle aged and was quite pleasant at first. There wasn't too much I could do at this point as I still had no feeling in my arm whatsoever. Actually, my arm was in a cuff sling and still felt like lead. I was wondering how I was going to exercise my arm when I couldn't even raise it. I was told to go to her in the morning and we would start rehabilitation on my arm.

I was resting in my room that afternoon when a nurse came to see me about my lunch and dinner arrangements. Tonight, I was to have dinner in my room, but tomorrow I was told that I would be picked up with a wheelchair and escorted to the dining room with the other patients to have all my main meals from now on. I didn't like this idea. I liked eating in the privacy of my own room. I didn't have any choice in the matter. Those were the rules, so who was I to make a fuss?

I would oblige. At least I could have breakfast, in my room. Dinner was served at 5.30pm. It took a while to eat my food, I still was getting used to eating left-handed, and I was only able to open half my mouth. This is the main reason for preferring my privacy. After dinner I watched a little television before retiring for the evening.

The next day started off with breakfast at 6am, then showered and dressed by 8am. I still didn't like help in this area, by the nurse or even my husband. There are situations that arrive in life I found, where having to deal through areas out of your comfort zone can indeed be very difficult to manage. This for me was one of these areas. I hated being washed by someone else and believe me I made it known. It was only about a week later when I was placed in the shower and left for five minutes to try to wash myself.

Then, a nurse would come back and help me only if I asked her. I learned to dress myself with my left hand only. I must admit it took me a long time to dress myself and to learn to put a ponytail in my hair, but the main challenge for me was applying make-up.

It is amazing what you are capable of doing when you are forced into a situation that's out of your control. I have learned to become ambidextrous. This is a talent having a stroke has forced me to engage.

I recall being asked by one of the councillors to meet her in her office. She said she had a short video for me to watch that would be extremely beneficial for me. It was going to help me when I returned home. So, I went as

I was a little curious about this video. As I sat in my wheelchair in her office, the councillor began by telling me how sorry she was for me. I couldn't help but think, "what was there to be sorry about?"

Then the video started. It was about a man and a woman that had both had strokes and how their daily chores were done a little different now, such as the way they bathed and dressed themselves, dressing the stroke side first, to the way they would walk, eat, socialize and so forth.

I felt so sorry for these two people on the video that it brought tears to my eyes. But I never felt connected. I never felt that it was relevant to me. I didn't feel the connection and wondered why I was watching this film.

The councillor looked at me for a while, then wrote a few notes and then asked me a question. The question was. Did I see the comparison to the people in the video and myself? I straight away said "NO". This question really made me upset. I didn't view myself like these people in the video. I wasn't well, I knew that, but I couldn't look like that, could I? Do I look like those poor souls on the video? It hit me like a ton of bricks. That woman in the video was me!

I sat in my chair for quite some time and just sobbed. The councillor squatted down beside me and said, "We need to talk about a few things. How you're going to cope at home, things that you'll find difficult now, such as making the bed, hanging out the washing, preparing dinner, going shopping and so forth. Have you thought of any of these things?"

As I sat there sobbing, I just shook my head. I hadn't really placed much thought on my life changing. I thought life was going to return to the way it was before. Really, I never contemplated my life being different. I just thought in a few weeks I would make a full recovery. I had to! Then I started to think, "What if I don't? "

I began to feel very afraid. I was afraid of not knowing what my future had in store for me.

I was staring reality in the face, and I didn't like what I saw. The video was a wakeup call and now I was truly awake. Many thoughts were flooding through my mind, too many for me to cope with at once. I just wanted to get out of that room and go back to mine. I felt safe there. I needed to be left alone for a while with my own thoughts.

As I laid on my bed that video kept playing through my mind. I was trying to imagine my life stuck in this wheelchair, but as hard as I tried I couldn't. Something inside me said, "I'll be alright and not to worry. I was going to leave this hospital on my two feet. I kept seeing myself walking and I knew in my heart it was going to be a reality for me."

The next time I saw my husband I tried to relay the way I was feeling but I would get so upset because I couldn't express myself properly. My brain and mouth were on two very different paths. The frustration I felt at this particular time of my life I would never wish upon anyone. I am not a very patient person. I found this to be extremely hard for me, overwhelmingly challenging. But as challenging as I thought I had it, it was nothing compared to what some of the other patients that I got acquainted with, had to go through. It didn't take long for me to realize how fortunate I really was. I was able to experience this firsthand and met some lovely people in Wyong Hospital. I still think of these people today and wonder how they are doing.

There was an elderly gentleman in particular that I came to admire in hospital. He had just become an amputee, but also had a mild stroke. He treated me like a granddaughter. The first time I met him was at my first visit to the dining room. It was the middle of January 1993, and it was a very hot summer.

I had just been wheeled in and was asked where I wanted to sit. As I looked around the room, I became very unsettled as they were mainly stroke victims there. They looked very scary to me and many of them were drooling and looked extremely disfigured. (Of course, I didn't realize that I looked the same.)

Anyway, I then heard a voice from the back of the room "Come over here, we need pretty young blood at this table." I looked over and saw an elderly gentleman with one leg in a wheelchair and a big grin on his face. Then the nurse wheeled me over to his table and from that day onwards I ate at the same table every day.

That man loved to tell stories of the adventures he had lived through in his lifetime. He told me funny stories and sad stories, but he had a fantastic zest for life and was a real fighter. He loved his family. He made me forget where I was for a brief moment. He could see the uncomfortable look on my face when I glanced around the room to see these poor elderly patients not able to feed themselves, some of them not even knowing where they were and denying the other half of their body. Some of them would cry out that they wanted to go home, and some wanted to know why their family hadn't come to see them. It was a little overwhelming for me, I had never seen this before, but the elderly gentleman made dining time bearable.

I sometimes would see him when I had to go to physiotherapy. I thought I had it hard. This poor man had lost his leg due to having diabetes. At least I still had my two legs. I never complained again during my sessions. I remember a poem I read in hospital about a man wishing for a new pair of shoes and another man wishing for feet so he could wear shoes. It prioritizes everything for you, doesn't it?

As well as the amputee, there was another quite friendly chap that sat at the dining table. He was a big man, around 6 feet 2, and about 140 kilos. He had a stroke as well and had already been in hospital for 3 months. He was very nice too but didn't say much. I don't think he was handling the stroke very well. He didn't appear to get many visitors. I would see him down at physiotherapy. He was struggling with his walking.

I remember one time he was left between two steel bars, and he called out to his therapist for help. The therapist took a little time getting back to him. In the meantime, the poor chap had wet himself. I felt so sorry for him. He was so embarrassed.

He looked at me – I just gave him a smile and said, "It happens, don't worry."

You see a lot of things you wouldn't normally see when you're staying in a rehab unit. There are a lot of people suffering that you're just not aware of. Staying in this unit opened my eyes. We tend to take life for granted. Especially the little things, such as walking and talking. We don't give it a second thought, but you do when it's been taken away from you.

I recall going to the Occupational Therapist for sessions concerning my right arm and hand. Normally you don't have to think about picking up an object – it happens automatically. Well, it used to for me too, but now I had to think about moving my fingers. Looking at them, I was really concentrating hard on trying to make them move. Do you know I sat there for 30 minutes every day with the Occupational Therapist trying to move a finger?

The first time a moved my small finger was not while I stayed in the hospital, it was when I had become an outpatient. It was 7 months and 3 days since the date of my stroke. That's how long it took my brain to make new pathways. It was one of the most memorable days of my life. I would go 3 times a week to get electric pulses rushed through my arm and hand. I remember changing therapists because the one I originally had told me after only one month (because nothing was happening yet) to get used to doing everything with my left hand because I would never get use of my right hand again. I remember being devastated and ringing my husband up crying.

My husband then arranged for me to see another Occupational Therapist and she was great. She was only in her twenties, but she was very knowledgeable and had great ideas and techniques for her young age. She became very important to me during and after my stay at Wyong Hospital. Even though it took a long time for movement to come back to my hand, she assured me that it would. When I first moved my little finger, I knew then that I had finally connected new pathways from my brain regarding my arm and hand, and that eventually I would regain movement in every finger, which eventually I did.

Time was passing slowly for me in hospital. I couldn't wait for the day when I could return home. My husband and children would come to see me nearly every day. I knew my husband wanted me home too.

During one of my family's visits my two boys, being boys aged 8 and 4, decided to go exploring up and down my corridor where they came across an elderly lady that had lost both of her legs. For some reason they found this amusing and started to laugh at her. When my husband realized what they were laughing about he took them aside had a serious talk to them. The elderly lady had heard our boy's laugh at her and for this reason my husband took our two boys to see this elderly lady and apologise to her, also giving her a bunch of flowers and a small gift. The lady was deeply moved, and our boys were genuinely sorry. From that day on our boy's would pop in to see the lady when they would come to visit me.

They learned a valuable lesson.

Days had turned into weeks. The hospital was starting to feel like home to me. My days consisted of mainly therapy, but I also had free time. I was starting to feel like I was away at camp, as I couldn't remember the last time I had to do any housework. It is going to feel strange I thought, when I do leave here, and my routine will be completely different.

Lunch time was my favourite part of the day. It was straight after lunch that I had free time. I would be taken to the garden outside my room along with my new friends. We would then have coffee and cake and listen to the elderly gentleman's stories. I felt a connection to these patients somehow.

I didn't realize at the time that I was slowly changing. I didn't realize that the stroke was altering my personality. I felt more comfortable with these people than my own family. I guess it was because these people were going through similar things as I was. I didn't feel like they were comparing me to the way I was before the stroke because they didn't know me then. They weren't looking at me with pity or focusing on my appearance. They just saw me and enjoyed my company. They didn't have unrealistic expectations of me, so I could relax and just be myself.

I had up and down days. I would sometimes laugh and sometimes cry. Not always knowing why. My emotions were scrambled all over the place and I couldn't explain it. My husband caught the biggest beating from my emotions. Sometimes he would only stay for 20 minutes and then would go home because I somehow made him upset with me. He said that I had changed and wanted his wife back. As you can imagine this would upset me as I felt like I was still the same person. I felt a lot of pressure from my husband in this area. I knew he still loved me. I also knew he was going through a hard time trying to cope with his wife having a stroke. He didn't like change, but then I never asked to be in this situation either. I knew there was going to be an adjusting period when I returned home. I was prepared for this.

It must be hard to see someone you love going through an experience like this. One day your partner is healthy and then another day they're not. I had to try to see my situation through my husband's eyes. He was a man who liked everything just so. He was a perfectionist and liked to be in total control. I suppose he must have felt helpless and

frustrated that he couldn't fix this situation I
was in. He wasn't used to that and that made
him extremely anxious. He was also really
scared that my feelings for him would
change.

I guess he didn't know what to expect. There
was now an area of uncertainty in his life that
he never thought he would ever have to deal
with. He told me it wasn't just me that had a
stroke, the whole family had a stroke. He
seemed to think I was a little self-absorbed.

Maybe I was, I don't know. I just wanted to
concentrate on getting better, for myself and
for my family.

There was one evening I had an experience I
would never forget. I had gone to bed and

was watching television when an elderly man entered my room. I had never seen him before and, at first, I thought he had entered my room by mistake. He called me Margaret. He obviously had the wrong room. He began to walk towards me still calling me Margaret. He was getting a little frantic and said we had to hurry to catch the next train.

I then realized this man was suffering from Alzheimer's disease. He was starting to get annoyed with me because I wasn't responding to his request. I couldn't speak very well all I could say was "Please go away" as I reached for the buzzer that was attached to my bed. I rang it 3 times before a nurse finally came. I was so relieved to see her as he was trying to get into my bed, stating his undying love for me. He honestly thought I was Margaret. (I gathered that Margaret must have been his wife.)

As the nurse escorted the elderly man back to his room, the nurse turned to me and said she would come back and see me as soon as her patient was back in bed.

While she was gone, I realized I was more shaken up than I thought. For the first time I felt insecure with myself. I mean, I couldn't run away, which was the first instinctive reaction you have. I couldn't get out of my bed, and I still couldn't walk. Then I thought to myself, what if the man became violent with me, I couldn't even protect myself. I began to sob a little. I was angry with myself, even though I knew it wasn't my fault that I couldn't walk. I had to try harder. I never wanted to be in this situation again. I had to be able to walk and protect myself.

The nurse entered my room about 20 minutes later and apologized about her patient. She told me he was suffering from the recent passing of his wife. He also had Alzheimer's disease, like I suspected. The nurse was going to put him in another ward in the morning, and for my safety the nurse locked my door for the evening.

I felt sorry for the elderly man – how alone must he feel? It got me thinking how fragile we really are, and that we should never take our loved ones for granted, or our health. All of a sudden, I longed to see my family and to tell them how much I loved and needed them.

The next morning it was business as usual. I was putting more time into my walking physio. I was starting to make improvements in this area, which I was proud of. I could walk down the whole length between the two steel posts. This was a great accomplishment for me. I could even make it to the dining room if I had a nurse supporting an arm each. I was however as slow as a snail, and I couldn't run a marathon, but I was making forward progress.

I hoped I would be well enough to go home soon.

Before too long Dr Crimmins came to see me at Wyong Hospital to see how I was getting on. He was pleasantly surprised with my progress, but he said I still had a long way to go. He was going to get my Occupational Therapist to go to my home to see about altering things to make my life easier for me when I would return home. He said that he would like me to go home weekends at first to see how I was able to cope. During the week I would still be staying in hospital. It was likened to a trial, or adjustment period. I was happy with that.

The Occupational Therapist did go to my home. She was very concerned about the steps into my home. I had 5 steps out the front of my house and 13 at the back. There was also my bathroom. It had to be fitted out with some handles for me to be able to support myself when I was able to stand in the shower and it also needed handles around the bathtub. There were other small adjustments that needed to be done before they would even consider me coming home for the weekend.

As we lived in Governmental Housing, my husband had to put these alterations in writing to get permission for these adjustments. These adjustments took a few weeks and then the Occupational Therapist went back to investigate. I was finally given the ok to come home for my first weekend visit. I was ecstatic.

I told the patients about my prospect of going

home during my free time, they were all

happy for me.

A LIGHT AT THE END OF THE TUNNEL

It was finally Saturday. I was to go home for the weekend after breakfast to spend the night at my home and return to Wyong Hospital for dinner Sunday. I was excited to go home but also a little anxious.

As my husband came to get me, I was surprised with the emotions that I was experiencing. I got a little teary. I was taken out of the hospital by wheelchair. It was still going to be a while until I was going to be able to walk out, but that was a goal I had firmly fixed in my head.

When we arrived at the car my children were all there waiting for me. They were happy to see me. As we drove home the children all had things to tell me. My youngest daughter had made me a welcome home card.

It wasn't long before we had arrived home. As we entered the driveway, I got a flash of me leaving in the ambulance. It was a very strange sensation. I had to compose myself before I attempted to get out of the car.

My husband told the children to go inside first as he had to help me get inside. I was given a forked stick to help me walk and my husband supported my stroke side. It took about 15 minutes for me to get inside. I wanted to walk inside all on my own but that was a bit ambitious at this stage. It was going to take several weeks to accomplish this task.

I remember getting inside my home when for a second, I wasn't paying attention to my taking steps. You see, I really had to concentrate while I was learning to walk again. I had to think of the process of walking, by this I mean I couldn't just walk like I use to, I actually had to think with every step I made. Heel first then bend your knee and flow through to the ball of your foot and repeat. It was exhausting this was one of these areas that I use to take for granted. Anyway, I lost my footing and tripped over on my lounge room floor.

My family naturally rushed to my aid. I was totally embarrassed. My husband helped me to the lounge. There was an awkward silence for a moment. It dawned on me that life for me was going to take major adjustment.

It was strange sitting in my lounge room, I felt like a visitor in my own home. I was told by my family to rest, and they would get anything I needed. I knew they were feeling a little anxious too. It had been quite a while since I was home. It would be awkward for all of us for a while.

My husband went to the kitchen to prepare lunch. He brought lunch to me on a tray into the lounge room. The children went and ate their lunch in the dining room.

After lunch the children gave me some presents that they had made themselves. I still have them today. I still didn't talk too much – my family did most of the talking. There wasn't too much I could do. I got tired really easily. I laid down on the lounge for a couple of hours. My children weren't used to seeing me like this, I was always on the go, but those days were gone.

We had a quiet afternoon, sitting at home just watching television. I told my husband I didn't want any visitors yet, even though I knew I had family and friends that wanted to see me. I wasn't ready for being on exhibition yet. That's how I was feeling at that moment. It would take me time to feel comfortable in the presence of people again, how long, I really couldn't say.

My brother rang my home to ask my husband how I was doing (I am extremely close to my brother). He had gone overseas with his wife prior to me having the stroke. He was also going to visit our mother as well (she had moved to Germany in 1986). They were all deeply concerned for my heath. My mother has since moved to Queensland and has been there for the past 10 years. We see each other twice a year and have a very special bond.

My mother-in-law rang as well. She wanted to come up and stay with us when I returned home for good, which I didn't mind. I was going to need all the help I could get. I had to keep telling myself this because I needed help now even though it was very difficult for me to accept. I had always been self-sufficient, so relying on other people's help was not going to be easy for me.

It was approaching dinner time, and the atmosphere was a little awkward for me. These were the same people that I knew in this house, yet something was very different. Everybody was trying too hard. My husband wouldn't let me do anything for myself, and the children were just too quiet. My children and I had a good relationship, but I noticed a little difference in each one of them. I couldn't put my finger on it at the time, but it did feel different.

Maybe it was just me, but they appeared to look and talk to me differently. My daughters were still very loving and very helpful, but they looked at me with scared concerned eyes. I wanted to take that away from them. My eldest son didn't come too close to me. In fact, he never hugged me again. My youngest son was still my baby.

I felt strange sensations being back in my home and as much as I wanted to be there with my husband and children, there was a big part of me that wanted to go back to the hospital. I kept asking myself. "What's wrong with me?"

Before too long my husband had prepared dinner, my daughters had set the table. I was escorted to the table with help from my husband. After prayer, my family started to eat their dinner when my eldest son noticed that I was eating with an unusual utensil and wanted to know why.

The utensil was a knife and fork in one. Since I was only able to use one hand my Occupational Therapist arranged this utensil for me as well as other gadgets to make life easier for me around the house. My husband explained this to our children. They understood.

After dinner I was taken straight back to the lounge room. I felt so bad that I couldn't help to clean up the kitchen. I laid down and watched some more television. It was about

30 minutes when the rest of the family came to join me. I couldn't help but notice that my youngest daughter was very quiet, and she kept staring at me. Later I found out why.

It turns out my daughter thought that the hospital had cloned me. Yes, she actually thought that the hospital found someone who looked like me and they sent that someone to my family while the real me was getting better in hospital. Can you imagine how scared she must have felt? It saddens me every time I think of that.

I was feeling tired and wanted to go to bed. The children said good night to me and my husband, yet again, helped me. I lay down on my bed and dozed off to sleep straight away, only to wake up one hour later. I had been reliving the night of my stroke in my dreams and was extremely distressed. My husband didn't get any sleep that night. He held me in his arms all night long. He would say repeatedly, "I've got you now, its ok. I'll take good care of you. I love you Shell." I couldn't help but wonder if I'd ever be able to sleep in my bed without reliving the stroke. Only time would tell. I needed my husband's reassurance.

The next day came and went and before I knew it, I was going back to Wyong Hospital. I continued the weekend visits for a few weeks. I needed to be home permanently though, as it was taking its toll on my family, particularly my husband, as he had returned to work, and was finding it hard juggling taking the children to school, going to work, going home, preparing meals, keeping up with the housework, and visiting me as well. He had been doing this for several months and just wanted our life back.

I was only allowed to go home if I became an Outpatient. I would miss my new friends that I acquired during my long stay in the hospital, but my deepest desire was to be home with my family. I felt that I needed their support and was missing them terribly. I thought I had been in hospital long enough and could continue the rest of my progress from home. I was starting to feel anxious for my husband as he had never been apart from me before. Neither had my children.

Being an outpatient, I had the best of both worlds. I would be home with my family, which would eliminate a lot of stress, as well as concentrating on my recovery.

As an outpatient I had to go back to the hospital 3 times a week for 2-hour sessions so I could continue progressing with my rehabilitation. I was to do this for as long as it took. I agreed and I did go for rehabilitation on and off for years after that, this was the only way I would regain some of my former self. It kept me physically and mentally strong, though it was a definite challenge.

I remember my last morning tea in Wyong Hospital we were all progressing health wise rather well. We were a great support to each other. We were all going to be outpatients for a while and wanted to keep up with each other's progress. Before too long we said our goodbyes and were off on our own.

I recall my first day back at home. My children had made a big banner that went right across the lounge room wall, it said, "Welcome Home Mummy" It naturally touched my heart.

Yes, I was back! I thought I could just pick up where I left off. It wasn't as easy as that.

My family adjusted to my condition better than I did. They wanted to do everything for me. My eldest son used humour to help. As for me, I just became angry and frustrated with myself. I was very stubborn to say the least. I resented help from anybody, which was stupid I know. I just wanted to do the things that I use to do, like simple household chores such as making the bed, washing and hanging up the clothes, going grocery shopping and so forth. Instead, I had family and friends doing these things for me.

Watching other people clean my house, iron my clothes, vacuum, mop the floor and cook my family dinner made me feel utterly useless. I had to fight the urge to criticize the quality of their help, as being a perfectionist was still in me. I wanted everything to be 'just so', but I couldn't do it myself. My brain was still working but my body was far behind it.

Would I ever be back to normal?

I would try to walk around the house without the aid of my walking stick. I could manage by holding or grabbing onto furniture. I was also determined to be able to get back into cleaning my own house.

I remember making the bed with one arm. Tucking the sheets in can be terribly difficult with one arm, so can hanging up clothes on the line. Since I only had the use of one arm, I had to invent a new technique for hanging up washing. It was likened to a juggling act when I hung up the clothes. I incorporated my teeth to add pegs to achieve this.

It's amazing what ideas you come up with to substitute the use of your limbs when they don't work. I found all sorts of ways to clean my house, though I didn't have nearly as much energy as I used to. I would have to lie down for an hour or so whenever I attempted to clean or do anything around the house.

THE LEARNING CURVE NEVER ENDS

My stubbornness and my determination to try to get back to normal put me back into hospital a few months later. I even underwent counselling to help me in accepting my new limitations. My body was thoroughly exhausted. I had to learn that I couldn't clean like I use to, my limitations were different now and I had to learn to accept this. I stayed in the hospital for a week, then I returned home with strict instructions to accept help.

My in-laws decided to stay with us for a week. This was my mother-in-law's request. I was to have a babysitter, as my husband didn't trust me not to do anything when I returned home. He knew me too well and was worried that I wouldn't be able to break old habits. I didn't mind though. I was really exhausted, and I knew it would put my husband's mind at ease that someone was with me at all times. So, the in-laws came to stay.

I must say it was nice to have company for that week. The children had never been with their grandparents for that amount of time before. My mother-in-law was known for her Italian dishes, and she would cook up a storm. My husband appreciated this immensely. I imagine he liked the break and now could relax a little after work, though my daughters were a great help – my husband had great support from my daughters as we did train them very well in this area.

As time went on, we quickly adapted to a new routine where the bulk of the burden was on my husband's shoulders. As I mentioned before he worked at Wyong Hospital, which was great for us, being in the situation we now found ourselves in.

My husband was able to start work a little later so as to help get the children ready for school and he was able to take me to rehab as well as popping in to check up on me a few times throughout the day to make sure I was alright. This gave him great comfort as he was the biggest worrywart you've ever seen. He was trying hard to cope the best way he could.

My husband never really accepted my stroke. He would often cry in bed. Even to this day he has been heard to say that he wishes he could have his 'old' Shell back, which is hard for me to take. He doesn't realise how that hurts.

The stroke had happened to all of us, and our life was never the same again. It has put our marriage to the test and put unnecessary strain on our family. Our family has gone through good and bad times. We have never had an abundance of wealth. That was never important to us. We lived a simple life, and we were always there for each other at any time, day or night.

I often feel guilty that I couldn't do certain things with my children due to my health, but I did always love them and I'm sure they knew that. I'm sorry that this experience caused them any insecurity. I'm sorry that they had to grow up a little sooner than they should have, particularly my girls. I'm sorry that over the past few years I went into deep depression.

It has been a major struggle, but at the end of the day we have to look at the positives we have in this life. It is easy to feel sorry for yourself, but where does that get you?

I have learned a great deal from this stroke. I have learned that you find out who your friends are, and that I have more empathy for people, given their situation. You sometimes have to accept help from different people, no matter how hard it is for you. You should be aware that you should never take the ones you love for granted. That is so easy to do.

My husband and I would have many arguments about this subject. He would say that I was so focused on getting better and doing it all on my own that he felt that I didn't appreciate him and was pushing him away rather than getting closer to him. I'm sorry for that.

We don't know what each day will bring, so it makes sense that we make each day the best it can be. That is one of the main reasons why I've tried to resolve any major issues with anyone I care about. Life's too short to hold any hard feelings or grudges.

I have come to see that people can be cruel in this life. I recall being down at my local shopping centre for the first time after months of rehabilitation. I remember walking through the shopping centre with my neighbour. I was walking along with my stick, when I overheard people whispering and laughing at the way I walked. I recall seeing my own reflection in the windows of the stores not recognizing that the disabled figure I saw was indeed me. I looked and I saw a reflection unrecognizable to me. I have cried many tears over the last few years but fortunately I have learned to accept myself and I am doing ok.

My children all grew up and they have their own lives now with their partners. My husband and I see our children regularly as they didn't move too far from home. We ended up moving 10 years ago as the house we were living in was too hard for me with all the steps. We moved into a new home that had no steps and was close to transport and the shops.

I never learned to drive; I didn't have the reflexes. Instead, I learned to walk everywhere.

My youngest daughter ended up becoming my care giver at the age of 16, as I stated before. We have a very special bond, as I do with all my children. My husband is still working for Wyong Hospital.

As for me, life is still a constant struggle. I developed quite a few ailments since my stroke, including Fibromyalgia Syndrome (FMS) Chronic Fatigue Syndrome (CFS) as well as Arthritis and bouts of depression. I have learned to deal with all of them and take life one day at a time.

I am a survivor and I know that I'm not alone – there are many people in this world going through worse things than me. I congratulate these people. Keep your fighting spirit!

I believe the mind is a strong tool. You've heard the saying 'mind over matter' – I believe that to be true.

When I went to see Dr Crimmins for my yearly check-up after the stroke, he just gasped when he saw me walk into his office. He said I was living proof of having strong determination and a strong mind. He said I actually willed myself well. He couldn't believe how far I had progressed, health wise. He also said my prognosis wasn't very good the last time he saw me, but I've proved to the doctors (him included) that anything is possible when you put your mind to it. I am a survivor and being stubborn turned out to be a blessing for me.

He asked my permission to tell my story as he was going to speak at a seminar in Queensland. I just laughed and said "sure, if it will help anyone, I'd be honoured."

This is where I'll end my reflections within my mind. I tell it with truth and sincerity and most of all, love for my family, without them I wouldn't have had the inspiration or determination to fight for my life. I thank them.

THE END

A NOTE FROM THE AUTHOR

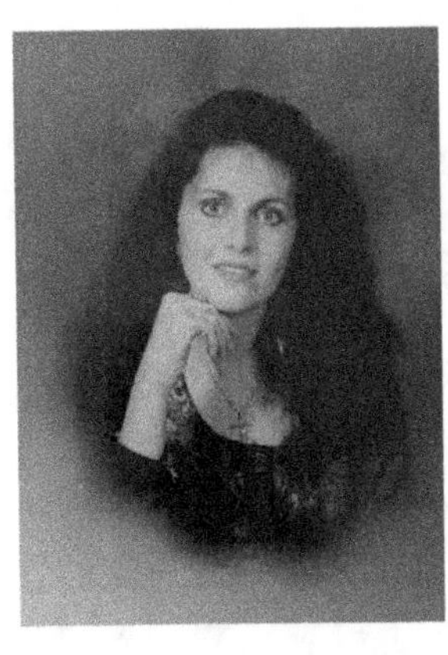

This my real-life experience as a stroke survivor. I hope it will help other victims of stroke to know there is light at the other end.

Never give up. Where there's life there's hope.